Renal Diet Tasty Recipes

50 Tasty and Incredible Recipes to Enjoy Your Diet

Elisabeth Peterson

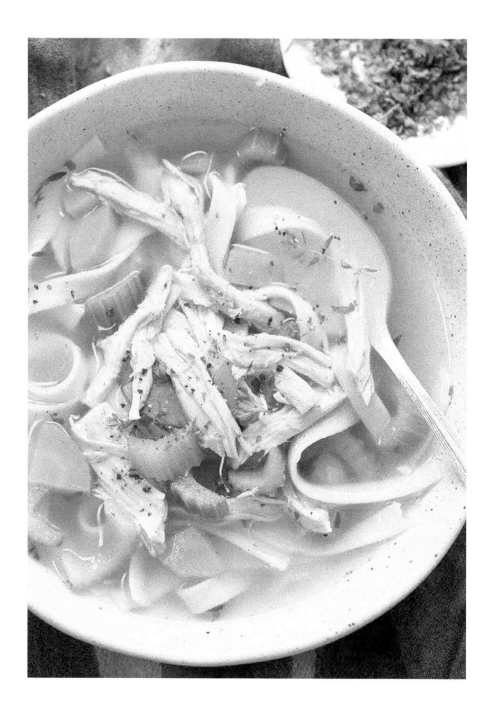

© **Copyright 2021 - All rights reserved.**

The content contained within this book may not be reproduced, duplicated or transmitted without direct written permission from the author or the publisher.

Under no circumstances will any blame or legal responsibility be held against the publisher, or author, for any damages, reparation, or monetary loss due to the information contained within this book. Either directly or indirectly.

Legal Notice:

This book is copyright protected. This book is only for personal use. You cannot amend, distribute, sell, use, quote or paraphrase any part, or the content within this book, without the consent of the author or publisher.

Disclaimer Notice:

Please note the information contained within this document is for educational and entertainment purposes only. All effort has been executed to present accurate, up to date, and reliable, complete information. No warranties of any kind are declared or implied. Readers acknowledge that the author is not engaging in the rendering of legal, financial, medical or professional advice. The content within this book has been derived from various sources. Please consult a licensed professional before attempting any techniques outlined in this book.

By reading this document, the reader agrees that under no circumstances is the author responsible for any losses, direct or indirect, which are incurred as a result of the use of information contained within this document, including, but not limited to, — errors, omissions, or inaccuracies.

Table of Contents

Peach High-Protein Smoothie 7

Strawberry Fruit Smoothie 8

Cranberry Smoothie 10

Berry Cucumber Smoothie 12

Raspberry Peach Smoothie 13

Power-Boosting Smoothie 15

Chili Tofu Noodles 16

Curried Cauliflower 18

Elegant Veggie Tortillas 20

Simple Broccoli Stir-fry 22

Braised Cabbage 24

Sautéed Green Beans 26

Penne Pasta with Asparagus 28

Garlic Mashed Potatoes 30

Cauliflower and Potato Curry 32

White Bean Veggie Burgers 34

Spinach Falafel Wrap 36

Spicy Tofu and Broccoli Stir-fry 38

Vegetable Biryani 41

Collard and Rice Stuffed Red Peppers 44

Stuffed Delicata Squash Boats with Bulgur and Vegetables 47

Barley and Roasted Vegetable Bowl.. 49

French Onion Soup 51

Cream of Watercress Soup 53

Curried Cauliflower Soup... 55

Roasted Red Pepper and Eggplant Soup 57

Traditional Chicken-vegetable Soup.. 59

Turkey and Lemon-grass Soup... 61

Herbed Soup with Black Beans 63

Tofu Soup.. 65

Turkey-bulgur Soup 67

Mediterranean Vegetable Soup 69

Onion Soup 71

Roasted Red Pepper Soup 73

Ground Beef and Rice Soup.. 75

Red Pepper and Brie Soup.. 77

Herbed Cabbage Stew 79

Paprika Pork Soup... 81

Winter Chicken Stew 83

Creamy Pumpkin Soup 85

Roasted Beef Stew.. 87

Spring Vegetable Soup 90

Leek and Carrot Soup 92

Spaghetti Squash and Yellow Bell-Pepper Soup 94

Steakhouse Soup 96

Cauliflower Soup 98

Kidney Diet Friendly Chicken Noodle Soup 100

Renal-friendly Cream of Mushroom Soup 102

Rotisserie Chicken Noodle Soup 104

Quick and Easy Ground Beef Soup 106

Peach High-Protein Smoothie

Preparation Time: 5 minutes

Cooking Time: 10 Minutes

Servings: 1

Ingredients:

- 1/2 cup ice
- 2 tablespoon powdered egg whites
- 3/4 cup fresh peaches
- 1 tablespoon sugar

Directions:

1. Set all the ingredients in a blender jug.
2. Give it a pulse for 30 seconds until blended well.
3. Serve chilled and fresh.

Nutrition Facts Per Serving:

Calories: 132kcal

Protein: 10 g

Fat: 0 g

Cholesterol: 0 mg

Potassium: 353 mg

Calcium: 9 mg

Fiber: 1.9 g

Strawberry Fruit Smoothie

Preparation Time: 5 minutes

Cooking Time: 10 Minutes

Servings: 1

Ingredients:

- 3/4 cup fresh strawberries
- 1/2 cup liquid pasteurized egg whites
- 1/2 cup ice
- 1 tablespoon brown sugar

Directions:

1. Set all the ingredients in a blender jug.
2. Give it a pulse for 30 seconds until blended well.
3. Serve chilled and fresh.

Nutrition Facts Per Serving:

Calories: 156 kcal

Protein: 14 g

Fat: 0 g

Cholesterol: 0 mg

Potassium: 400 mg

Phosphorus: 49 mg

Calcium: 29 mg

Fiber: 2.5 g

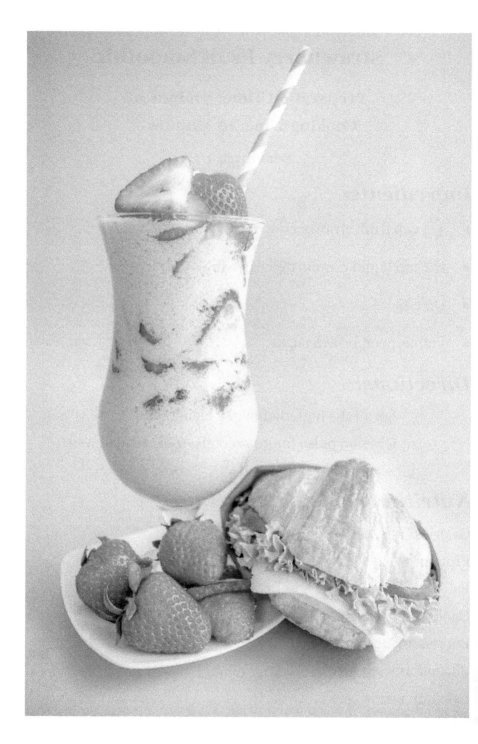

Cranberry Smoothie

Preparation Time: 5 minutes
Cooking Time: 10 Minutes
Servings: 1

Ingredients:

- 1 cup frozen cranberries
- 1 medium cucumber, peeled and sliced
- 1 stalk of celery
- Handful of parsley
- A squeeze of lime juice

Directions:

1. Set all the ingredients in a blender jug.
2. Give it a pulse for 30 seconds until blended well.
3. Serve chilled and fresh.

Nutrition Facts Per Serving:

Calories: 42 kcal

Protein: 12 g

Fat: 0.03 g

Cholesterol: 0 mg

Potassium: 220 mg

Phosphorus: 34mg
Calcium: 19 mg
Fiber: 1.4 g

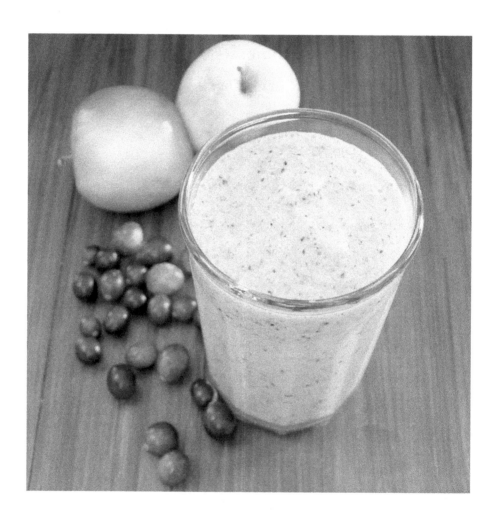

Berry Cucumber Smoothie

Preparation Time: 10 minutes
Cooking Time: 5 Minutes
Servings: 1

Ingredients:

- 1 medium cucumber, peeled and sliced
- 1/2 cup fresh blueberries
- 1/2 cup fresh or frozen strawberries
- 1/2 cup unsweetened rice milk
- Stevia, to taste

Directions:

1. Set all the ingredients in a blender jug.
2. Give it a pulse for 30 seconds until blended well.
3. Serve chilled and fresh.

Nutrition Facts Per Serving:

Calories: 76 kcal

Protein: 1 g

Carbohydrates: 15 g

Fat: 0 g

Sodium: 113 mg

Potassium: 230 mg

Phosphorus: 37 g

Raspberry Peach Smoothie

Preparation Time: 5 minutes

Cooking Time: 3 Minutes

Servings: 2

Ingredients:

- 1 cup frozen raspberries
- 1 medium peach, pit removed, sliced
- 1/2 cup silken tofu
- 1 tablespoon honey
- 1 cup unsweetened vanilla almond milk

Directions:

1. Set all the ingredients in a blender jug.
2. Give it a pulse for 30 seconds until blended well.
3. Serve chilled and fresh.

Nutrition Facts Per Serving:

Calories: 132 kcal

Protein: 3.5 g

Carbohydrates: 14 g

Sodium: 112 mg

Potassium: 310 mg

Phosphorus: 63 mg

Calcium: 32 mg

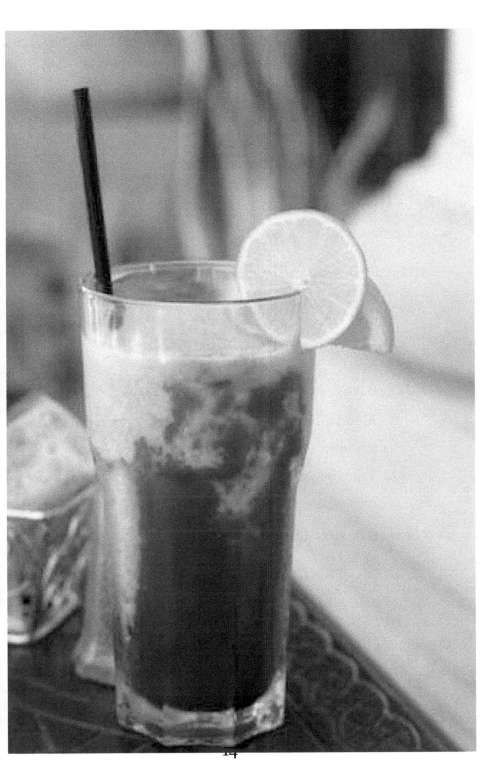

Power-Boosting Smoothie

Preparation Time: 5 minutes
Cooking Time: 10 Minutes
Servings: 2

Ingredients:

- 1/2 cup water
- 1/2 cup non-dairy whipped topping
- 2 scoops whey protein powder
- 1 1/2 cups frozen blueberries

Directions:

1. Blend all ingredients using a blender and pulse till smooth.
2. Transfer into 2 serving glasses and serve immediately.

Nutrition Facts Per Serving:

Calories: 190 kcal
Fat: 7 g
Carbohydrates: 23.8 g
Protein: 23.2 g
Potassium: 263 mg
Sodium: 106 mg
Phosphorus: 30 mg

Chili Tofu Noodles

Preparation time: 5 minutes
Cooking time: 50 minutes
Servings: 4

Ingredients:

- 1/2 diced red chili
- 1 cup rice noodles
- 1/2 juiced lime
- 6 ounces pressed and cubed silken firm tofu
- 1 teaspoon grated fresh ginger
- 1 tablespoon coconut oil
- 1 cup green beans
- 1 minced garlic clove

Directions:

1. Steam the green beans for 10-12 minutes or according to package directions and drain.
2. Cook the noodles in a pot of boiling water for 10-15 minutes or according to package directions.
3. Meanwhile, heat a wok or skillet on a high heat and add coconut oil.

4. Now add the tofu, chili flakes, garlic and ginger and sauté for 5-10 minutes.
5. After doing that, drain in the noodles along with the green beans and lime juice then add it to the wok.
6. Toss to coat.
7. Serve hot!

Nutrition Facts Per Serving:

Calories 313 kcal

Protein: 10 g

Carbs: 28 g

Fat: 12 g

Sodium: 99 mg

Potassium: 312 mg

Phosphorus: 120 mg

Curried Cauliflower

Preparation time: 5 minutes
Cooking time: 25 minutes
Servings: 4

Ingredients:

- 1 teaspoon turmeric
- 1 diced onion
- 1 tablespoon chopped fresh cilantro
- 1 teaspoon cumin
- 1/2 diced chili
- 1/2 cup water
- 1 minced garlic clove
- 1 tablespoon coconut oil
- 1 teaspoon garam masala
- 2 cups cauliflower florets

Directions:

1. Attach the oil to a skillet on medium heat.
2. Sauté the onion and garlic for 5 minutes until soft.

3. Add in the cumin, turmeric and garam masala and stir to release the aromas.
4. Now add the chili to the pan along with the cauliflower.
5. Stir to coat.
6. Pour in the water and reduce the heat to a simmer for 15 minutes.
7. Garnish with cilantro to serve.

Nutrition Facts Per Serving:

Calories: 133 kcal

Protein: 2 g

Carbs: 11 g

Fat: 7 g

Sodium: 35 mg

Potassium: 328 mg

Phosphorus: 39 mg

Elegant Veggie Tortillas

Preparation time: 30 minutes
Cooking time: 30 minutes
Servings: 12

Ingredients:

- 1/2 cup of chopped broccoli florets
- 1 1/2 cups of chopped cauliflower florets
- 1 tablespoon of water
- 2 teaspoon of canola oil
- 1 1/2 cups of chopped onion
- 1 minced garlic clove
- 2 tablespoons of finely chopped fresh parsley
- 1/2 cup of low-cholesterol liquid egg substitute
- Freshly ground black pepper, to taste
- 4 (6-inches) warmed corn tortillas

Directions:

1. In a microwave bowl, place broccoli, cauliflower and water and microwave, covered for about 3-5 minutes.
2. Remove from the microwave and drain any liquid.

3. Heat oil on medium heat.
4. Add onion and sauté for about 4-5 minutes.
5. Add garlic and then sauté it for about 1 minute.
6. Stir in broccoli, cauliflower, parsley, egg substitute and black pepper.
7. Reduce the heat and let it simmer for about 10 minutes.
8. Detach from heat and keep aside to cool slightly.
9. Place broccoli mixture over 1/4 of each tortilla.
10. Fold the outside edges inward and roll up like a burrito.
11. Secure each tortilla with toothpicks to secure the filling.
12. Cut each tortilla in half and serve.

Nutrition Facts Per Serving:

Calories: 539.19 kcal

Fat: 11.86 g

Carbs: 96.49 g

Protein: 8.1 g

Fiber: 6.3 g

Potassium: 950 mg

Sodium: 219.29 mg

Phosphorus: 600 mg

Simple Broccoli Stir-fry

Preparation time: 40 minutes
Cooking time: 15 minutes
Servings: 4

Ingredients:

- 1 tablespoon of olive oil
- 1 minced garlic clove
- 2 cups of broccoli florets
- 2 tablespoons of water

Directions:

1. Heat oil on medium heat.
2. Add garlic and then sauté for about 1 minute.
3. Attach the broccoli and stir fry for about 2 minutes.
4. Stir in water and stir fry for about 4-5 minutes.
5. Serve warm.

Nutrition Facts Per Serving:

Calories: 89 kcal

Fat: 3.6 g

Carbs: 3.3 g

Protein: 1.3 g

Fiber: 1.2 g

Potassium: 230 mg

Sodium: 23 mg

Phosphorus: 49 mg

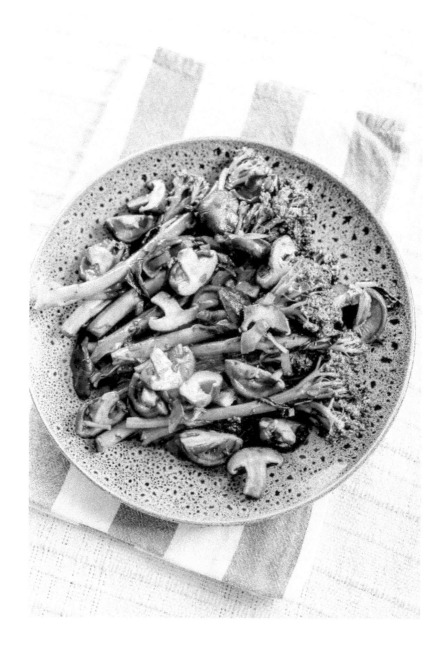

Braised Cabbage

Preparation time: 30 minutes
Cooking time: 40 minutes
Servings: 4

Ingredients:

- 1 1/2 teaspoon of olive oil
- 2 minced garlic cloves
- 1 thinly sliced onion
- 3 cups of chopped green cabbage
- 1 cup of low-sodium vegetable broth
- Freshly ground black pepper, to taste

Directions:

1. In a large skillet, warm oil on medium-high heat.
2. Add garlic and then sauté for about 1 minute.
3. Add onion and sauté for about 4-5 minutes.
4. Add cabbage and sauté for about 3-4 minutes.
5. Stir in broth and black pepper and immediately, reduce the heat to low.
6. Cook, covered for about 20 minutes
7. Serve warm.

Nutrition Facts Per Serving:

Calories: 99 kcal

Fat: 1.8 g

Carbs: 6.6 g

Protein: 1.1 g

Fiber: 1.9 g

Potassium: 600 mg

Sodium: 99 mg

Phosphorus: 39 mg

Sautéed Green Beans

Preparation Time: 10 minutes
Cooking Time: 30 minutes
Servings: 4

Ingredients:

- 2 cup frozen green beans
- 1/2 cup red bell pepper
- 2 tsp. margarine
- 1/4 cup onion
- 1 tsp. dried dill weed
- 1 tsp. dried parsley
- 1/4 tsp. black pepper

Directions:

1. Cook green beans in a large pan of boiling water until tender, then drain.
2. While the beans are cooking, melt the margarine in a skillet and fry the other vegetables.
3. Add the beans to sautéed vegetables.
4. Sprinkle with freshly ground pepper and serve with meat and fish dishes.

Nutrition Facts Per Serving:

Calories: 130 kcal

Fat: 7 g

Carbs: 8 g

Protein: 4 g

Sodium: 76 mg

Potassium: 340 mg

Phosphorus: 55 mg

Penne Pasta with Asparagus

Preparation Time: 30 minutes
Cooking Time: 10 minutes
Servings: 4

Ingredients:

- 2 tbsp. unsalted butter
- 1 clove of garlic
- 1 tsp. red pepper
- 1 tsp. black pepper
- 1cup asparagus, cut into 2-inch pieces
- 2 tsp. lemon juice
- 4 cup whole wheat penne pasta, cooked
- 1/4 cup shredded cheddar cheese
- 1/4 tsp. Tabasco hot sauce

Directions:

1. Add unsalted butter in a skillet over medium heat.
2. Fry garlic and red pepper flakes for 2-3 minutes.
3. Add asparagus, Tabasco sauce, lemon juice, and black pepper to skillet and cook for a further 6 minutes.

4. Add pre-cooked, hot pasta and cheese. Toss and serve.

Nutrition Facts Per Serving:

Calories: 387 kcal

Carbs: 49 g

Protein: 13 g

Sodium: 93 mg

Potassium: 258 mg

Phosphorous: 252 mg

Garlic Mashed Potatoes

Preparation Time: 5 minutes
Cooking Time: 25 minutes
Servings: 4

Ingredients:

- 2 medium potatoes, peeled and sliced
- 2 tbsp. unsalted butter
- 1/4 cup 1% low-fat milk
- 2 garlic cloves

Directions:

1. Double-boil or soak the potatoes to reduce potassium if you are on a low potassium diet.
2. Boil potatoes and garlic until soft for about 20 minutes. Drain.
3. Beat the potatoes and garlic with butter and milk until smooth.

Nutrition Facts Per Serving:

Calories: 168 kcal

Fat: 12g

Carbs: 29 g

Protein: 5 g

Sodium: 59 mg

Potassium: 189 mg

Phosphorous: 57 mg

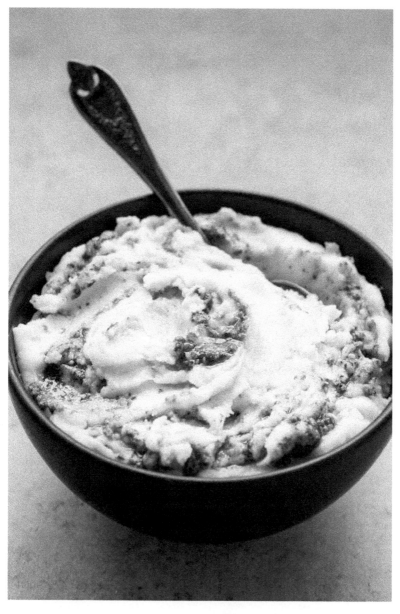

Cauliflower and Potato Curry

Preparation time: 40 minutes
Cooking time: 30minutes
Servings: 4

Ingredients:

- 2 tablespoons canola oil
- 1/2 sweet onion, chopped
- 2-inch piece ginger
- 3 garlic cloves, minced
- 1 teaspoon ground turmeric
- 1 teaspoon ground cumin
- 1 small head cauliflower, cut into florets
- 1 medium potato, diced
- 2 small tomatoes, diced
- 1 small green Chile, stemmed, seeded, and diced
- 1/2 cup water
- Juice of 1/2 lemon
- 1/4 cup chopped cilantro leaves
- 1 teaspoon garam masala

- ½ cup basmati rice or 1 whole wheat bread, for serving

Directions:

1. Warm up the olive oil. Add the onion and cook.
2. Attach the ginger and garlic, and cook until fragrant. Stir in the turmeric and cumin. Add the cauliflower, potato, tomatoes, Chile, and water. Bring to a simmer, reduce the heat, and cover.
3. Cook, stirring occasionally, for 25 minutes, until the potatoes and cauliflower are tender.
4. Stir in the lemon juice, cilantro, and garam masala. Serve over rice or with bread.

Nutrition Facts Per Serving:

Calories: 180 kcal

Total Fat: 7 g

Saturated Fat: 1 g

Cholesterol: 0 mg

Carbohydrates: 19 g

Fiber: 3 g

Protein: 3 g

Sodium: 20 mg

Phosphorus: 65 mg

Potassium: 546 mg

White Bean Veggie Burgers

Preparation time: 10 minutes
Cooking time: 25 minutes
Servings: 4

Ingredients:

- 1 cup canned white beans
- 1 cup cooked rice
- 1 teaspoon garlic powder
- 2 teaspoons dried thyme
- 1/2 teaspoon ground chipotle pepper
- 1/2 sweet onion, finely chopped
- 1/2 cup fresh or frozen corn
- 1/2 cup bell pepper
- Juice of 1 lemon
- 1/3 cup all-purpose flour
- 1 large egg
- Freshly ground black pepper
- 2 teaspoons extra-virgin olive oil

Directions:

1. In a large bowl, break the beans with a potato masher, leaving a few whole beans as desired. Attach the rice, garlic powder, thyme, chipotle pepper, onion, corn, bell pepper, lemon, flour, and egg, and merge well to blend. Sprinkle it with pepper.
2. With your hands, make the mixture into four patties.
3. In a skillet over medium heat, warm up the olive oil. Grill each burger. Serve.

Nutrition Facts Per Serving:

Calories: 401.27 kcal

Total Fat: 8.37 g

Carbs: 67.88 g

Protein: 16.33 g

Sodium: 410.43 mg

Potassium: 800 mg

Phosphorus: 240 mg

Spinach Falafel Wrap

Preparation time: 10 minutes
Cooking time: 15 minutes
Servings: 4

Ingredients:

- 6 ounces baby spinach
- 1 (15-ounce) can chickpeas, drained and rinsed
- 2 teaspoons ground cumin
- 3/4 cup flour
- 2 tablespoons canola oil, divided, for frying
- 1/4 cup plain, unsweetened yogurt
- 2 garlic cloves, minced
- Juice of 1 lemon
- Freshly ground black pepper
- 4 tortillas
- 1 cucumber, cut into spears
- 2 slices red onion
- Salad greens, for serving

Directions:

1. Set the spinach in a colander in the sink, and pour boiling water over it to wilt the spinach. Allow it to cool.
2. In a food processor, attach the spinach, chickpeas, cumin, and flour. Pulse until just blended.
3. Divide the mixture into tablespoon-size balls, and use your hands to press them flat into patties.
4. In a large skillet over medium-high heat, warm up 1 tablespoon of oil. Add half of the falafel patties, and cook for 2 to 3 minutes on each side, until browned and crisp. Repeat with the remaining falafel patties.
5. In a small bowl, combine the yogurt, garlic, lemon juice, and pepper.
6. On each tortilla, place 3 falafel patties, a couple cucumber spears, a few red-onion rings, and a handful of salad greens. Set each with 1 tablespoon of the yogurt sauce.

Nutrition Facts Per Serving:

Calories: 687.45 kcal

Total Fat: 21.76 g

Carbs: 108.63 g

Protein: 21.06 g

Sodium: 461.27 mg

Potassium: 900 mg

Phosphorus: 600 mg

Spicy Tofu and Broccoli Stir-fry

Preparation time: 15 minutes

Cooking time: 30 minutes

Servings: 4

Ingredients:

For the Sauce

- 3 garlic cloves
- 2-inch piece ginger, peeled
- 2 tablespoons honey
- 1/4 cup rice wine vinegar
- 2 tablespoons extra-virgin olive oil

For the Stir-Fry

- 1/2 package extra-firm tofu
- 1 cup long-grain white rice
- 2 tablespoons extra-virgin olive oil
- 1 cup chopped broccoli
- 1 cup shredded carrots
- 3 scallions, finely chopped

Directions:

To Make the Sauce
1. Combine the garlic, ginger, honey, vinegar, and olive oil in a food processor, and purée until smooth.

To Make the Stir-Fry
1. Divide the tofu into small cubes, and press the excess moisture from the tofu using paper towels, repeating several times until dry.
2. In a medium pot, cook the rice according to package directions for about 20 minutes.
3. In a large skillet over medium heat, warm up the olive oil. Add the tofu to the pan in a single layer. Carefully add one quarter of the sauce to the pan and continue to cook, flipping the tofu only once or twice every 4 minutes, until it is well browned. With a slotted spoon, transfer the tofu to a plate lined with paper towels to drain.
4. Add the broccoli to the pan. Cook, covered, stirring often, until fork-tender, about 5 minutes. Attach the carrots and continue to cook for an additional 3 minutes, until softened. Add the remaining sauce to the vegetables, return the tofu to the pan, and stir to mix. Garnish with scallions and serve over rice.

Nutrition Facts Per Serving:

Calories: 410 kcal
Total Fat: 18 g
Saturated Fat: 3 g

Cholesterol: 0 mg

Carbohydrates: 51 g

Fiber: 4 g

Protein: 13 g

Phosphorus: 222 mg

Potassium: 487 mg

Sodium: 51 mg

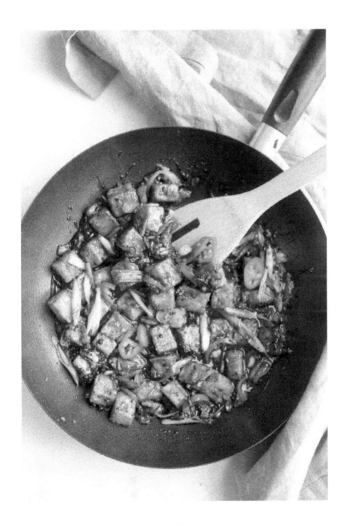

Vegetable Biryani

Preparation time: 10 minutes

Cooking time: 50 minutes

Servings: 4

Ingredients:

- 1 cup basmati rice
- 2 tablespoons olive oil or butter, divided
- 1/2 teaspoon curry powder
- 1/2 teaspoon cumin seeds
- 1/2 teaspoon coriander seeds
- 13/4 cups water plus 2/3 cup water, divided
- 1/2 sweet onion, chopped
- 2 garlic cloves, minced
- 1 teaspoon ground coriander
- 1/2 teaspoon ground cardamom
- 1/2 teaspoon ground cumin
- 1/4 teaspoon turmeric
- 1 cup cauliflower
- 1 cup green beans

- 1 carrot

- 1/4 cup chopped cilantro leaves

Directions:

1. In a small bowl, wash the rice until the water runs clear.
2. In a medium stockpot over medium heat, warm up 1 tablespoon of olive oil. Attach the curry powder, cumin seeds, and coriander seeds, stirring constantly, until fragrant, about 30 seconds. Attach the rice to the pot along with 1 3/4 cups of water. Set to a boil; reduce the heat, cover, and simmer for about 20 minutes.
3. In a skillet over medium heat, set the remaining tablespoon of olive oil. Add the onion, and cook for 6 to 8 minutes, until tender. Add the garlic and cook for an additional minute. Add the coriander, cardamom, cumin, and turmeric to the skillet, and stir constantly, toast until fragrant, about 1 minute. Add the cauliflower, beans, and carrots, stirring to coat, and cook for 2 to 3 minutes. Attach the remaining 2/3 cup of water to the pan, cover, and cook for 7 to 10 minutes, until the vegetables are just fork-tender.
4. Add the rice to the vegetables, and stir to blend. Serve topped with cilantro leaves.

Nutrition Facts Per Serving:

Calories: 470 kcal

Total Fat: 15.92 g

Saturated Fat: 1 g

Cholesterol: 4 mg

Carbohydrates: 74.39 g

Fiber: 3 g

Protein: 4 g

Phosphorus: 170 mg

Potassium: 500 mg

Sodium: 58.36 mg

Collard and Rice Stuffed Red Peppers

Preparation time: 10 minutes
Cooking time: 50 minutes
Servings: 4

Ingredients:

- 2 medium red bell peppers
- 2 tablespoons extra-virgin olive oil, divided
- Freshly ground black pepper
- 6 cups loosely packed collard greens, trimmed
- 1/2 sweet onion, chopped
- 3 garlic cloves, minced
- 1 cup cooked white rice or ½ cup basmati rice
- Juice of 1 lemon
- 1/4 cup toasted sunflower seeds, divided

Directions:

1. Preheat the oven to 400F.
2. Halve the peppers through the stems, and detach the seeds and stems. Garnish the inside and outside of the peppers with 1 tablespoon of olive oil and season

with the pepper. Place the peppers cut-side down in a baking dish.
3. Bake them for 10 to 15 minutes, until just tender. Remove from the oven and flip the peppers cut-side up. Set aside, leaving the oven on.
4. In a large saucepan, Set 4 cups of water to a boil. Add the collard greens and cook until just tender, 5 to 7 minutes. Drain and rinse under cold water. Chop finely.
5. In a large skillet, heat the remaining tablespoon of olive oil over medium heat. Add the onion, and cook, stirring often, for 5 to 7 minutes, until it begins to brown. Add the garlic and cook until fragrant. Stir in the collard greens. Detach from the heat, and stir in the cooked rice, half amount of sunflower seeds and lemon juice. Season with pepper.
6. Divide the filling between the pepper halves and top each pepper half with 1 tablespoon of the sunflower seeds.
7. Add 1/4 cup of water to the baking dish, cover with aluminum foil, and bake for 20 minutes, until heated through. Uncover and bake.

Nutrition Facts Per Serving:

Calories: 450 kcal
Total Fat: 9 g
Saturated Fat: 1 g

Cholesterol: 0 mg

Carbohydrates: 50 g

Fiber: 5 g

Protein: 8 g

Phosphorus: 147 mg

Potassium: 397 mg

Sodium: 20 mg

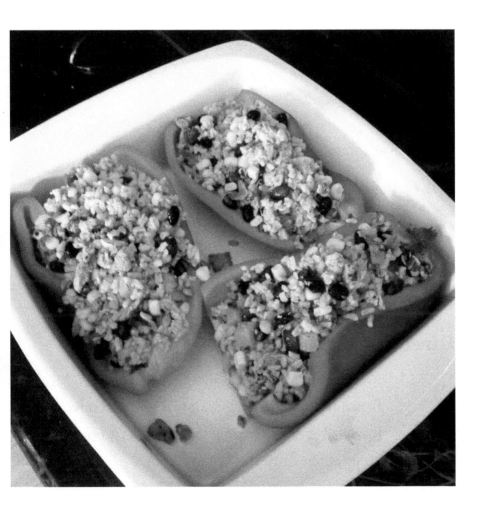

Stuffed Delicata Squash Boats with Bulgur and Vegetables

Preparation time: 10 minutes

Cooking time: 1 hour

Servings: 4

Ingredients:

- 2 small delicate squash, halved lengthwise and seeded
- 6 teaspoons extra-virgin olive oil, divided
- 1 cup bulgur
- 1/2 sweet onion, diced
- 2 tablespoons chili powder
- 1 cup canned black beans, drained and rinsed
- 1/2 cup frozen or fresh corn kernels
- 2 scallions, thinly sliced, for garnish

Directions:

1. Preheat the oven to 425F.
2. Brush the cut squash with 2 teaspoons of olive oil and place cut-side down on a baking sheet. Cook for 25 to 30 minutes, until the flesh is tender.

3. Meanwhile, in a saucepan, bring the bulgur and 2 cups of water to a boil. Lower the heat, covers, and simmers for 12 to 15 minutes, until the liquid is absorbed. Drain well.
4. In a large skillet, set the remaining 4 teaspoons of olive oil over medium heat. Cook the onion for 4 to 5 minutes, until it just starts to brown. Stir in the chili powder, black beans, and corn. Stir in the bulgur, and cook for an additional minute.
5. Divide the filling between the squash halves, sprinkle with scallions, and serve.

Nutrition Facts Per Serving:

Calories: 591.67 kcal

Total Fat: 17.1 g

Carbs: 103.16 g

Protein: 17.87 g

Sodium: 573.46 mg

Potassium: 700 mg

Phosphorus: 340 mg

Barley and Roasted Vegetable Bowl

Preparation time: 15 minutes

Cooking time: 1 hour

Servings: 4

Ingredients:

- 2 small Asian eggplants, diced
- 2 small zucchini, diced
- 1/2 red bell pepper, chopped
- 1/2 sweet onion, cut into wedges
- 2 tablespoons extra-virgin olive oil, divided
- Freshly ground black pepper
- 1 cup barley
- Juice of 1 lemon
- 3 garlic cloves, minced
- 1/4 cup basil leaves, roughly chopped
- 1/4 cup crumbled feta cheese
- 2 cups arugula or mixed baby salad greens

Directions:

1. Preheat the oven to 425F.

2. In a medium bowl, toss the eggplant, zucchini, bell pepper, and onion with 1 tablespoon of olive oil, and arrange the vegetables in a single layer on a baking sheet. Season with pepper.
3. Roast the vegetables for about 25 minutes, stirring once or twice, until they are browned and tender. Set aside.
4. Meanwhile, in a medium pot, add the barley and 2 cups of water. Bring to a boil, reduce the heat to simmer, cover, and cook for 20 minutes. Turn off the heat, and let rest for 10 minutes. Fluff with a fork, and drain any remaining water.
5. In a small bowl, whisk the lemon juice, garlic, and remaining tablespoon of olive oil.
6. Toss the vegetables with the barley, and then mix together with the lemon-garlic dressing. Right before serving, stir in the basil, feta cheese, and salad greens.

Nutrition Facts Per Serving:

Calories: 447.62 kcal

Total Fat: 19.84 g

Carbs: 60.55 g

Protein: 12.9g

Sodium: 244 mg

Potassium: 880 mg

phosphorus: 230 mg

French Onion Soup

Preparation time: 10 minutes

Cooking time: 30 minutes

Servings: 5

Ingredients:

- 2 tablespoons unsalted butter
- 4 Vidalia onions, sliced thin
- 2 cups Easy Chicken Stock
- 2 cups water
- 1 tablespoon chopped fresh thyme
- Freshly ground black pepper

Directions:

1. Dissolve the butter.
2. Attach the onions to the saucepan and cook them slowly, stirring frequently, for about 10 minutes.
3. Attach the chicken stock and water, and bring the soup to a boil.
4. Reduce the heat to low and simmer the soup for 15 minutes.
5. Stir in the thyme and season the soup with pepper.
6. Serve piping hot.

Nutrition Facts Per Serving:

Calories: 120 kcal

Fat: 6 g

Carbohydrates: 7 g

Phosphorus: 22 mg

Potassium: 192 mg

Sodium: 57 mg

Protein: 2 g

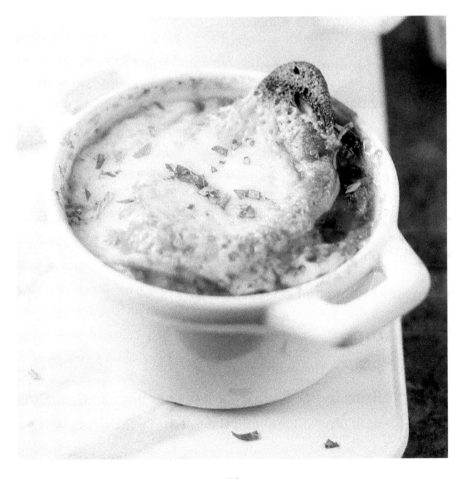

Cream of Watercress Soup

Preparation time: 15 minutes

Cooking time: 1 hour

Servings: 5

Ingredients:

- 6 garlic cloves
- 1/2 teaspoon olive oil
- 1 teaspoon unsalted butter
- 1/2 sweet onion, chopped
- 4 cups chopped watercress
- 1/4 cup chopped fresh parsley
- 3 cups water
- 1/4 cup lite cooking cream
- 1 tablespoon freshly squeezed lemon juice
- Freshly ground black pepper

Directions:

1. Preheat the oven to 400F.
2. Bring the garlic on a sheet of aluminum foil. Mizzle with olive oil and fold the foil into a little packet.

Place the packet in a pie plate and roast the garlic for about 20 minutes or until very soft.
3. Remove the garlic from the oven; set aside to cool.
4. In a large saucepan over medium-high heat, melt the butter. Sauté the onion for about 4 minutes or until soft. Add the watercress and parsley; sauté 5 minutes.
5. Stir in the water and roasted garlic pulp. Set the soup to a boil, and then reduce the heat to low.
6. Stew the soup for about 20 minutes or until the vegetables are soft.
7. Cool the soup for about 5 minutes, then purée in batches in a food processor along with the heavy cream.
8. Transfer the soup to the pot, and set over low heat until warmed through.
9. Add the lemon juice and season with pepper.

Nutrition Facts Per Serving:

Calories: 150 kcal

Fat: 8 g

Carbohydrates: 5 g

Sodium: 23 mg

Phosphorus: 46 mg

Potassium: 380 mg

Protein: 2 g

Curried Cauliflower Soup

Preparation time: 10 minutes

Cooking time: 40 minutes

Servings: 6

Ingredients:

- 1 teaspoon unsalted butter
- 1 small, sweet onion, chopped
- 2 teaspoons minced garlic
- 1 small head cauliflower
- 3 cups water
- 2 teaspoons curry powder
- 1/2 cup light sour cream
- 3 tablespoons chopped fresh cilantro

Directions:

1. In a large saucepan, warm up the butter over medium-high heat and sauté the onion and garlic for about 3 minutes or until softened.
2. Add the cauliflower, water, and curry powder.
3. Set the soup to a boil, and then reduce the heat to low and simmer.

4. Pour the soup into a food processor and purée until the soup is smooth and creamy (or use a large bowl and a handheld immersion blender).
5. Transfer the soup back into a saucepan and stir in the sour cream and cilantro.
6. Heat the soup on medium-low for about 5 minutes or until warmed through.

Nutrition Facts Per Serving:

Calories 196.2 kcal

Total Fat: 9.1g

Carbs: 24.77 g

Protein: 8.43 g

Sodium: 164.49 mg

Potassium: 900 mg

Phosphorus: 130 mg

Roasted Red Pepper and Eggplant Soup

Preparation time: 20 minutes
Cooking time: 40 minutes
Servings: 6

Ingredients:

- 1 small, sweet onion, cut into quarters
- 2 small red bell peppers, halved
- 2 cups cubed eggplant
- 2 garlic cloves, crushed
- 1 tablespoon olive oil
- 1 cup Easy Chicken Stock (here)
- Water
- 1/4 cup chopped fresh basil
- Freshly ground black pepper

Directions:

1. Preheat the oven to 350F.
2. Put the onions, red peppers, eggplant, and garlic in a large ovenproof baking dish.
3. Drizzle the vegetables with the olive oil.

4. Roast the vegetables.
5. Cool the vegetables slightly and remove the skin from the peppers.
6. Purée the vegetables in batches in a food processor (or in a large bowl, using a handheld immersion blender) with the chicken stock.
7. Transfer the soup to a medium pot and add enough water to reach the desired thickness. Heat the soup to a simmer and add the basil.
8. Season with pepper and serve.

Nutrition Facts Per Serving:

Calories: 280kcal

Fat: 2 g

Total Fat: 9.14 g

Carbs: 21.45 g

Sodium: 183.45 mg

Potassium: 600 mg

Phosphorus: 130 mg

Traditional Chicken-vegetable Soup

Preparation time: 20 minutes

Cooking time: 35 minutes

Servings: 6

Ingredients:

- 1 tablespoon unsalted butter
- 1/2 sweet onion, diced
- 2 teaspoons minced garlic
- 2 celery stalks, chopped
- 1 carrot, diced
- 1 cup chopped cooked chicken breast
- 1 cup Easy Chicken Stock (here)
- 4 cups water
- 1 teaspoon chopped fresh thyme
- Freshly ground black pepper
- 2 tablespoons chopped fresh parsley

Directions:

1. Dissolve the butter.
2. Simmer the onion and garlic until softened.

3. Put the celery, carrot, chicken, chicken stock, and water.
4. Set the soup to a boil until the vegetables are tender.
5. Attach the thyme; simmer the soup for 2 minutes.
6. Flavor with pepper and serve topped with parsley.

Nutrition Facts Per Serving:

Calories: 246.18 kcal

Fat: 13.67g

Carbohydrates: 2 g

Protein: 18.63 g

Sodium: 298.51 mg

Potassium: 550 mg

Phosphorus: 180 mg

Turkey and Lemon-grass Soup

Preparation Time: 5 minutes
Cooking Time: 40 minutes
Servings: 4

Ingredients:

- 1 fresh lime
- 1/4 cup fresh basil leaves
- 1 tbsp. cilantro
- 1 cup chestnuts
- 1 tbsp. coconut oil
- 1 thumb-size minced ginger piece
- 2 chopped scallions
- 1 finely chopped green chili
- 4oz. skinless and sliced turkey breasts
- 1 minced garlic clove, minced
- 1/2 finely sliced stick lemon-grass
- 1 chopped white onion, chopped
- 4 cups water

Directions:

1. Crush the lemon-grass, cilantro, chili, 1 tbsp. oil, and basil leaves in a blender or pestle and mortar to form a paste.
2. Heat a large pan/wok with 1 tbsp. olive oil on high heat.
3. Sauté the onions, garlic, and ginger until soft.
4. Add the turkey and brown each side for 4-5 minutes.
5. Add the broth and stir.
6. Now add the paste and stir.
7. Next, add the chestnuts, turn down the heat slightly, and simmer for 25-30 minutes or until the turkey is thoroughly cooked through.
8. Serve hot with the green onion sprinkled over the top.

Nutrition Facts Per Serving:

Calories 340.83kcal

Total Fat 12.76g

Carbs 42.11g

Protein: 15.63 g

Sodium: 49.97 mg

Potassium: 720 mg

Phosphorus: 210 mg

Herbed Soup with Black Beans

Preparation Time: 10 minutes

Cooking Time: 10 minutes

Servings: 4

Ingredients:

- 2 tbsp. tomato paste
- 1/3 cup Poland pepper, charred, peeled, seeded and chopped
- 2 cups vegetable stock
- 1/4 tsp. cumin
- 1/2 tsp. paprika
- 1/2 tsp. dried oregano
- 2 tsp. fresh garlic, minced
- 1 cup onion, small diced
- 1 tbsp. extra-virgin olive oil
- 1.5 oz can black beans

Directions:

1. On medium fire, place a soup pot and heat oil. Attach onion and sauté until translucent and soft, around 4-5 minutes. Add garlic, cook for 2 minutes.

2. Attach the rest of the ingredients and bring to a simmer. Once simmering, turn off the fire and transfer to a blender. Puree ingredients until smooth.

Nutrition Facts Per Serving:

Calories: 148.73 kcal

Total Fat: 7.69 g

Carbs: 18.13 g

Sugars: 7.08 g

Protein: 3.73 g

Sodium: 816.43 mg

Potassium: 440 mg

Phosphorus: 37 mg

Tofu Soup

Preparation Time: 5 minutes

Cooking Time: 10 minutes

Servings: 2

Ingredients:

- 1 tbsp. miso paste
- 1/8 cup cubed soft tofu
- 1 chopped green onion
- 1/4 cup sliced Shiitake mushrooms
- 3 cups Renali stock
- 1 tbsp. soy sauce

Directions:

1. Take a saucepan, pour the stock into this pan and let it boil on high heat. Reduce heat to medium and let this stock simmer. Add mushrooms to this stock and cook for almost 3 minutes.
2. Take a bowl and mix soy sauce (reduced salt) and miso paste together in this bowl. Add this mixture and tofu to stock. Simmer for nearly 5 minutes and serve with chopped green onion.

Nutrition Facts Per Serving:

Calories: 129 kcal

Fat 7.8 g

Sodium 484 mg

Potassium 435 mg

Protein: 11 g

Carbs: 5.5 g

Phosphorus: 73.2 mg

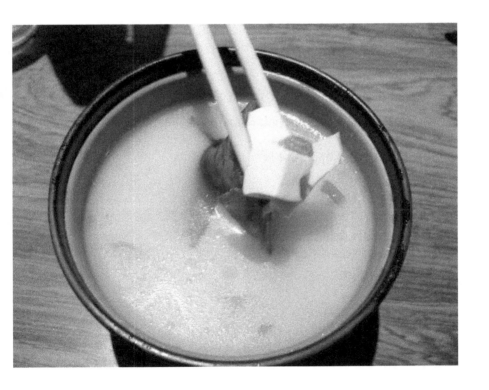

Turkey-bulgur Soup

Preparation time: 25 minutes
Cooking time: 45 minutes
Servings: 6

Ingredients:

- 1 teaspoon olive oil
- 2 oz. cooked ground turkey, 93% lean
- 1/2 sweet onion, chopped
- 1 teaspoon minced garlic
- 4 cups water
- 1 cup Easy Chicken Stock (here)
- 1 celery stalk, chopped
- 1 carrot, sliced thin
- 1/2 cup shredded green cabbage
- 1/2 cup bulgur
- 2 dried bay leaves
- 2 tablespoons chopped fresh parsley
- 1 teaspoon chopped fresh sage
- 1 teaspoon chopped fresh thyme

- Pinch red pepper flakes
- Freshly ground black pepper

Directions:

1. Heat the olive oil. Sauté the turkey until the meat is cooked through.
2. Attach the onion and garlic and sauté for about 3 minutes or until the vegetables are softened. Attach the water, chicken stock, celery, carrot, cabbage, bulgur, and bay leaves.
3. Set the soup to a boil and then reduce the heat to low and simmer until the bulgur and vegetables are tender.
4. Detach the bay leaves and stir in the parsley, sage, thyme, and red pepper flakes.
5. Season with pepper and serve.

Nutrition Facts Per Serving:

Calories: 277.93 kcal

Total Fat: 9.57 g

Carbs: 38.59 g

Protein: 11.91 g

Sodium: 259.82 mg

Potassium: 550 mg

Phosphorus: 160 mg

Mediterranean Vegetable Soup

Preparation Time: 5 minutes

Cooking Time: 30 minutes

Servings: 4

Ingredients:

- 1 tbsp. oregano
- 2 minced garlic cloves
- 1 tsp. black pepper
- 1 diced zucchini
- 1 cup diced eggplant
- 4 cups water
- 1 diced red pepper
- 1 tbsp. extra-virgin olive oil
- 1 diced red onion

Directions:

1. Soak the vegetables in warm water before use.
2. In a large pot, add the oil, chopped onion, and minced garlic.
3. Sweat for 5 minutes on low heat.

4. Add the other vegetables to the onions and cook for 7-8 minutes.
5. Add the stock to the pan and bring to a boil on high heat.
6. Stir in the herbs, reduce the heat, and simmer for a further 20 minutes or until thoroughly cooked through.
7. Season with pepper to serve.

Nutrition Facts Per Serving:

Calories: 152 kcal

Protein: 1 g

Carbs: 6 g

Fat: 3 g

Sodium 3 mg

Potassium 229 mg

Phosphorus: 45 mg

Onion Soup

Preparation Time: 15 minutes
Cooking Time: 45 minutes
Servings: 6

Ingredients:

- 2 tbsp. chicken stock
- 1 cup chopped shiitake mushrooms
- 1 tbsp. minced chives
- 3 tsps. beef bouillon
- 1 tsp. grated ginger root
- 1/2 chopped carrot
- 1 cup sliced Portobello mushrooms
- 1 chopped onion
- 1/2 chopped celery stalk
- 2 quarts' water
- 1/4 tsp. minced garlic

Directions:

1. Take a saucepan and combine carrot, onion, celery, garlic, mushrooms (some mushrooms), and ginger in this pan. Add water, beef bouillon, and chicken stock

to this pan. Put this pot on high heat and let it boil. Decrease flame to medium and cover this pan to cook for almost 45 minutes.
2. Put all remaining mushrooms in one separate pot. Once the boiling mixture is completely done, put one strainer over this new bowl with mushrooms and strain cooked soup in this pot over mushrooms. Discard solid-strained materials.
3. Serve delicious broth with yummy mushrooms in small bowls and sprinkle chives over each bowl.

Nutrition Facts Per Serving:

Calories: 90.58 kcal

Total Fat: 1.09 g

Carbs: 17.44 g

Protein: 6.27 g

Sodium: 77.54 mg

Potassium: 710 mg

Phosphorus: 210 mg

Roasted Red Pepper Soup

Preparation Time: 30 minutes
Cooking Time: 35 minutes
Servings: 4

Ingredients:

- 4 cups low-sodium chicken broth
- 3 red peppers
- 2 medium onions
- 3 tbsp. lemon juice
- 1 tbsp. finely minced lemon zest
- A pinch of cayenne pepper
- 1/4 tsp. cinnamon
- 1/2 cup finely minced fresh cilantro

Directions:

1. In a medium stockpot, consolidate each one of the fixings except for the cilantro and warmth to the point of boiling over excessive warm temperature. Diminish the warmth and stew, ordinarily secured, for around 30 minutes, till thickened. Cool marginally. Utilizing a hand blender or nourishment

processor, puree the soup. Include the cilantro and tenderly heat.

Nutrition Facts Per Serving:

Calories: 175.67 kcal

Total Fat: 3.62 g

Carbs: 29.32 g

Sugars: 13.54 g

Protein: 12.81 g

Sodium: 157.85 mg

Potassium: 1000 mg

Phosphorus: 200 mg

Ground Beef and Rice Soup

Preparation time: 15 minutes
Cooking time: 1 ¼ hours
Servings: 6

Ingredients:

- 2 oz. extra-lean ground beef
- 1/2 small, sweet onion, chopped
- 1 teaspoon minced garlic
- 2 cups water
- 1 cup homemade low-sodium beef broth
- 1/2 cup long-grain white rice, uncooked
- 1 celery stalk, chopped
- 1/2 cup fresh green beans
- 1 teaspoon chopped fresh thyme
- Freshly ground black pepper

Directions:

1. Cook beef. Sauté, stirring often, for about 6 minutes until the beef is completely browned.
2. Drain off the excess fat and add the onion and garlic to the saucepan.

3. Sauté the vegetables until they are softened for 5 minutes.
4. Add the water, beef broth, and celery and simmer for 40 minutes.
5. Add rice for another 20 minutes
6. Add the green beans and thyme and simmer for 3 minutes.
7. Remove the soup from the heat and season with pepper.

Nutrition Facts Per Serving:

Calories: 235.55 kcal

Total Fat: 1.93 g

Carbs: 42.09 g

Protein: 11.48 g

Sodium: 244.87 mg

Potassium: 340 mg

Phosphorus: 141 mg

Red Pepper and Brie Soup

Preparation Time: 10 minutes

Cooking Time: 35 minutes

Servings: 4

Ingredients:

- 1 tsp. paprika
- 1 tsp. cumin
- 1 chopped red onion
- 2 chopped garlic cloves
- 1/4 cup crumbled brie
- 2 tbsps. extra virgin olive oil
- 4 chopped red bell peppers
- 4 cups water

Directions:

1. Warmth the oil in a pot over medium heat.
2. Sweat the onions and peppers for 5 minutes.
3. Add the garlic cloves, cumin, and paprika and sauté for 3-4 minutes.
4. Add the water and allow to boil before turning the heat down to simmer for 30 minutes.
5. Detach from the heat and allow to cool slightly.

6. Put the mixture in a food processor and blend until smooth.
7. Pour into serving bowls and add the crumbled brie to the top with a little black pepper.
8. Enjoy!

Nutrition Facts Per Serving:

Calories: 152 kcal

Protein: 3 g

Carbs: 8 g

Fat: 11 g

Sodium: 66 mg

Potassium: 270 mg

Phosphorus: 207 mg

Herbed Cabbage Stew

Preparation time: 20 minutes
Cooking time: 35 minutes
Servings: 6

Ingredients:

- 1 teaspoon unsalted butter
- 1/2 large, sweet onion, chopped
- 1 teaspoon minced garlic
- 6 cups shredded green cabbage
- 3 celery stalks, chopped with the leafy tops
- 1 scallion, chopped
- 2 tablespoons chopped fresh parsley
- 2 tablespoons freshly squeezed lemon juice
- 1 tablespoon chopped fresh thyme
- 1 teaspoon chopped savory
- 1 teaspoon chopped fresh oregano
- Water
- 1 cup fresh green beans
- Freshly ground black pepper

Directions:

1. In a medium stockpot over medium-high heat, dissolve the butter.
2. Sauté the onion and garlic in the melted butter for about 3 minutes or until the vegetables are softened.
3. Add the cabbage, celery, scallion, parsley, lemon juice, thyme, savory, and oregano to the pot, and pour enough water to cover the vegetables by about 4 inches.
4. Set the soup to a boil, reduce the heat to low, and simmer the soup for 10 minutes until the vegetables are tender.
5. Add the green beans and simmer for 3 minutes.
6. Season with pepper.

Nutrition Facts Per Serving:

Calories: 107.65 kcal

Total Fat: 2.42 g

Carbs: 21.19 g

Sugars: 10.47 g

Protein: 4.21 g

Sodium: 104.94 mg

Potassium: 680 mg

Phosphorus: 90 mg

Paprika Pork Soup

Preparation Time: 5 minutes

Cooking Time: 35 minutes

Servings: 2

Ingredients:

- 4 oz. sliced pork loin
- 1 tsp. black pepper
- 2 minced garlic cloves
- 3 cups water
- 1 tbsp. extra-virgin olive oil
- 1 chopped onion
- 1 tbsp. paprika

Directions:

1. In a large pot, attach the oil, chopped onion, and minced garlic.
2. Sauté for 5 minutes on low heat.
3. Add the pork slices to the onions and cook for 7-8 minutes or until browned.
4. Add the water to the pan and bring to a boil on high heat.
5. Season with pepper to serve.

Nutrition Facts Per Serving:

Calories: 250 kcal

Protein: 13 g

Carbs: 10 g

Fat: 9 g

Sodium: 269 mg

Potassium: 486 mg

Phosphorus: 158 mg

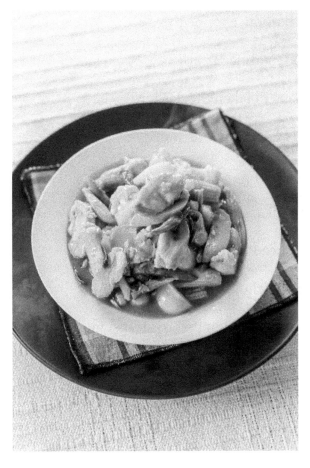

Winter Chicken Stew

Preparation time: 20 minutes

Cooking time: 50 minutes

Servings: 6

Ingredients:

- 1 tablespoon olive oil
- 1-pound boneless chicken
- 1/2 sweet onion, chopped
- 1 tablespoon minced garlic
- 2 cups Easy Chicken Stock (here)
- 1 cup plus 2 tablespoons water
- 1 carrot, sliced
- 2 celery stalks, sliced
- 1 turnip, sliced thin
- 1 tablespoon chopped fresh thyme
- 1 teaspoon finely chopped fresh rosemary
- 2 teaspoons cornstarch
- Freshly ground black pepper

Directions:

1. Heat the olive oil.
2. Sauté the chicken for about 6 minutes or until it is lightly browned, stirring often.
3. Attach the onion and garlic and sauté for 3 minutes.
4. Add the chicken stock, 1 cup water, carrot, celery, and turnip and bring the stew to a boil.
5. Set the heat to low and simmer or until the chicken is cooked through and tender for about 30 minutes.
6. Add the thyme and rosemary and simmer for 3 more minutes.
7. In a small bowl, toss together the 2 tablespoons of water and the cornstarch, and add the mixture to the stew.
8. Stir to incorporate the cornstarch mixture and cook for 3 to 4 minutes or until the stew thickens.
9. Detach from the heat and season with pepper.

Nutrition Facts Per Serving:

Calories: 482.34 kcal

Total Fat: 16.21 g

Carbs: 22.35 g

Protein 58.49g

Sodium: 566.84 mg

Potassium: 1371.32 mg

Phosphorus: 560 mg

Creamy Pumpkin Soup

Preparation Time: 10 minutes
Cooking Time: 20 minutes
Servings: 4

Ingredients:

- 1 onion, chopped
- 1 slice of bacon
- 2 tsp. ground ginger
- 1 tsp. cinnamon
- 1 cup applesauce
- 3 1/2 cups low sodium chicken broth
- 1.5 oz canned pumpkin
- Pepper to taste
- 1/2 cup light sour cream

Directions:

1. On medium-high fire, place a soup pot and add bacon once hot. Sauté until crispy, around 4 minutes. Discard bacon fat before continuing to cook. Add ginger, applesauce, chicken broth, and pumpkin.

Lightly season with pepper. Set to a simmer and cook for 11 minutes. Taste and adjust seasoning. Turn off fire, stir in sour cream and mix well.

Nutrition Facts Per Serving:

Calories: 320.91

Fat: 14.01 g

Fiber: 10 g

Carbs: 36 g

Protein: 10 g

Sodium: 262.9 mg

Potassium: 700 mg

Phosphorus: 200 mg

Roasted Beef Stew

Preparation time: 30 minutes
Cooking time: 1 ½ hour
Servings: 6

Ingredients:

- 1/4 cup all-purpose flour
- 1 teaspoon freshly ground black pepper
- Pinch cayenne pepper
- 1/2-pound boneless beef
- 2 tablespoons olive oil
- 1/2 sweet onion, chopped
- 2 teaspoons minced garlic
- 1 cup homemade beef stock
- 1 cup plus 2 tablespoons water
- 1 carrot, cut into 1/2-inch chunks
- 2 celery stalks, chopped with greens
- 1 teaspoon chopped fresh thyme
- 1 teaspoon cornstarch

- 2 tablespoons chopped fresh parsley

Directions:

1. Preheat the oven to 350F.
2. Set the flour, black pepper, and cayenne pepper in a large plastic freezer bag and toss to merge.
3. Attach the beef chunks to the bag and toss to season.
4. Heat the olive oil.
5. Sauté the beef chunks until they are lightly browned for about 10 minutes.
6. Detach the beef from the pot and set aside on a plate.
7. Attach the onion and garlic to the pot and sauté.
8. Attach 1 cup water, the beef drippings on the plate, the carrot, celery, and thyme.
9. Seal the pot tightly with a lid or aluminum foil and place in the oven.
10. Bake the stew until the meat is very tender for about 1 hour.
11. Flavor the stew with black pepper and serve topped with parsley.

Nutrition Facts Per Serving:

Calories: 392.73 kcal

Total Fat: 21.55 g

Carbs: 22.47 g

Protein: 28.31 g

Sodium: 407.68 mg

Potassium: 900 mg
Phosphorus: 310 mg

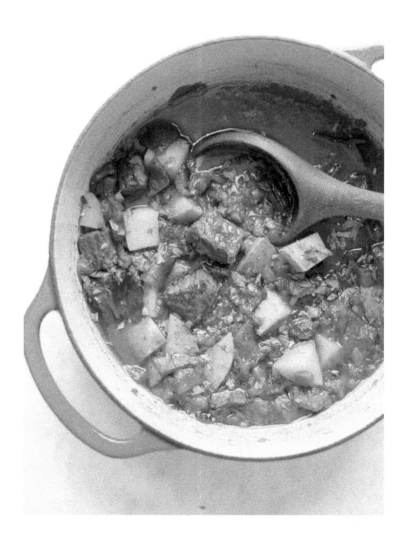

Spring Vegetable Soup

Preparation Time: 10 minutes

Cooking Time: 1 hour

Servings: 4

Ingredients:

- Vegetable broth (low-sodium): 4 cups
- Fresh green beans: 1 cup
- Half cup carrots
- Celery: 3/4 cup
- Garlic powder: 1 teaspoon
- Half cup onion
- Half cup mushrooms
- Olive oil: 2 tablespoons
- Dried oregano leaves: 1 teaspoon
- 1/4 teaspoon salt
- Half cup frozen corn

Directions:

1. Trim the green beans and chop into two-inch pieces
2. Chop up the vegetables.

3. In a pot, heat olive oil, sauté the onion and celery till tender.
4. Then add the remaining ingredients with the broth.
5. Let it boil and cook for about 40 minutes.
6. Lower the heat and let it simmer. Then serve.

Nutrition Facts Per Serving:

Calories: 144 kcal

Protein: 2 g

Carbohydrates: 13 g

Fat: 6 g

Sodium: 262 mg

Potassium: 365 mg

Phosphorus: 108 mg

Calcium: 48 mg

Fiber: 3.4 g

Leek and Carrot Soup

Preparation Time: 15 minutes
Cooking Time: 25 minutes
Servings: 4

Ingredients:

- leek
- 3/4 cup diced and boiled carrots
- 1 garlic clove
- 1 tbsp olive oil
- Crushed pepper to taste
- cups low sodium chicken stock
- Chopped parsley for garnish
- 1 bay leaf
- 1/4 tsp. ground cumin

Directions:

1. Trim off and take away a portion of the coarse inexperienced portions of the leek. At that factor, reduce daintily and flush altogether in water. Channel properly. Warmth the oil in an extensively based pot.

Include the leek and garlic, and sear over low warmth for two-3 minutes, till sensitive. Include the inventory, inlet leaf, cumin, and pepper.
2. Warmth the mixture to the point of boiling, mixing constantly. Include carrots and stew for 13 minutes. Modify the flavoring, eliminate the inlet leaf, and serve sprinkled with slashed parsley. To make a pureed soup, manner the soup in a blender or nourishment processor till smooth. Come again to the pan. Include 1/2 field milk. Bring to bubble and stew for 4 minutes.

Nutrition Facts Per Serving:

Calories 119.6kcal

Total Fat 7.48g

Carbs 12.41g

Sugars 4.47g

Protein 1.88g

Sodium 112.65mg

potassium 250mg

phosphorus 37mg

Spaghetti Squash and Yellow Bell-Pepper Soup

Preparation Time: 10 minutes
Cooking Time: 45 minutes
Servings: 4

Ingredients:

- 2 diced yellow bell peppers
- 2 chopped large garlic cloves
- 1 peeled and cubed spaghetti squash
- 1 quartered and sliced onion
- 1 tbsp. dried thyme
- 1 tbsp. coconut oil
- 1 tsp. curry powder
- 4 cups water

Directions:

1. Warmth the oil over medium-high heat before sweating the onions and garlic for 3-4 minutes.
2. Sprinkle over the curry powder.
3. Attach the stock and bring to a boil over a high heat before adding the squash, pepper, and thyme.

4. Turn down the heat, cover, and allow to simmer for 25-30 minutes.
5. Continue to simmer until squash is soft if needed.
6. Allow cooling before blitzing in a blender/food processor until smooth.
7. Serve!

Nutrition Facts Per Serving:

Calories: 150 kcal

Protein: 2 g

Carbs: 17 g

Fat: 4 g

Sodium: 32 mg

Potassium: 365 mg

Phosphorus: 50 mg

Steakhouse Soup

Preparation Time: 15 minutes
Cooking Time: 25 minutes
Servings: 4

Ingredients:

- 2 tbsps. soy sauce
- 2 boneless and cubed chicken breast halves
- 1/4 lb. halved and trimmed snow peas
- 1 tbsp. minced ginger root
- 1 minced garlic clove
- 1 cup water
- 2 chopped green onions
- 3 cups chicken stock
- 1 chopped carrot
- 3 sliced mushrooms

Directions:

1. Take a pot and combine ginger, water, chicken stock, Soy sauce (reduced salt), and garlic in this pot. Let them boil on medium heat, mix in chicken pieces,

and let them simmer on low heat for almost 15 minutes to tender chicken.
2. Stir in carrot and snow peas and simmer for almost 5 minutes. Add mushrooms to this blend and continue cooking to tender vegetables for nearly 3 minutes. Mix in the chopped onion and serve hot.

Nutrition Facts Per Serving:

Calories: 319 kcal

Carbs: 14 g

Fat: 15 g

Potassium: 225 mg

Protein: 29 g

Sodium: 389 mg

Phosphorous: 190 mg

Cauliflower Soup

Preparation Time: 5 minutes
Cooking Time: 30 minutes
Servings: 6

Ingredients:

- 1 teaspoon unsalted butter
- 1 small, chopped, sweet onion–
- 2 teaspoons minced garlic
- 1 small head cauliflower, cut into small florets
- 2 teaspoons curry powder
- Water to cover the cauliflower
- 1/2 cup light sour cream
- 3 tablespoons chopped fresh cilantro

Directions:

1. In a large saucepan, warm up the butter over medium-high heat and sauté the onion-garlic for about 3 minutes or until softened.
2. Add the cauliflower, water, and curry powder.

3. Set the soup to a boil, then reduce the heat to low and simmer for 20 minutes or until the cauliflower is tender.
4. Puree the soup until creamy and smooth with a hand mixer.
5. Transfer the soup back into a saucepan and stir in the sour cream and cilantro.
6. Warm the soup on medium heat for 5 minutes or until warmed through.

Nutrition Facts Per Serving:

Calories: 195.85 kcal

Total Fat: 9.09 g

Carbs: 24.71 g

Protein: 8.4 g

Sodium: 156.9 mg

Potassium: 1009 mg

Phosphorus: 190 mg

Kidney Diet Friendly Chicken Noodle Soup

Preparation Time: 10 minutes
Cooking Time: 25 minutes
Servings: 4

Ingredients:

- 1 cup cooked Chicken Breast
- Unsalted Butter: 1 tbsp.
- 1/2 cup of Chopped Celery
- Chicken Stock: 5 cups
- 1/2 tsp. Ground Basil
- 1/2 cup of chopped Onions
- Ground Black Pepper 1/4 tsp.
- Egg Noodles: 1 cup, Dry
- Sliced Carrots: 1 cup
- 1/2 tsp. Ground Oregano

Directions:

1. Chop up all the vegetables.
2. In a Dutch oven (5 quarts), melt butter over low heat.

3. Cook celery and onion for five minutes. Add in the carrots, oregano, chicken stock, basil, pepper, chicken and noodles.
4. Let it boil for 10 minutes.
5. Serve hot.

Nutrition Facts Per Serving:

Calories: 479.41 kcal

Total Fat: 17.49 g

Carbs: 51.84 g

Protein: 27.74 g

Sodium: 953.01 mg

Potassium: 1100 mg

Phosphorus: 370 mg

Renal-friendly Cream of Mushroom Soup

Preparation Time: 5 minutes
Cooking Time: 15 minutes

Servings: 2

Ingredients:

- Minced mushrooms: 1/4 cup
- Unsalted butter: 3 tbsp.
- All-purpose flour: 2 and a half tbsp.
- Sea salt, pepper to taste
- Low sodium chicken broth: half cup
- Finely chopped onion: 1/4 cup
- Unsweetened almond milk: half cup

Directions:

1. In a skillet, dissolve the butter and sauté onions till tender
2. Add mushrooms and cook for five minutes. Add flour and cook for 1 minute and stir for frying
3. Add in milk and broth mix continuously.
4. Let it simmer until it becomes thick for five minutes.

Nutrition Facts Per Serving:

Calories: 191 kcal
Total Fat: 18.2 g
Cholesterol: 45.8 mg
Sodium: 162.8 mg
Carbohydrates: 10.2 g
Dietary Fiber: 0.9 g
Protein: 2.1 g
Iron: 1 mg
Potassium: 123.7 mg

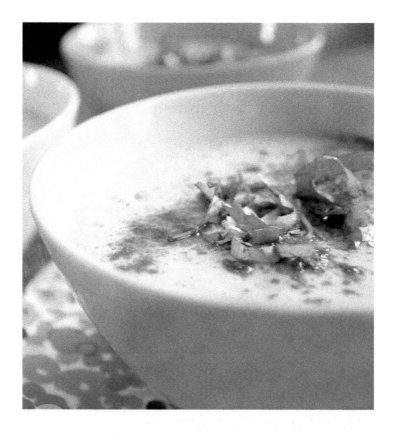

Rotisserie Chicken Noodle Soup

Preparation Time: 10 minutes
Cooking Time: 15 minutes
Servings: 2

Ingredients:

- Carrots: 1 cup, sliced
- 2 cups cooked rotisserie chicken
- 1/2 cup of onion, chopped
- Celery: 1 cup, sliced
- Chicken broth (low-sodium): 4 cups
- Fresh parsley: 3 tablespoons
- Wide noodles: 6 ounces, uncooked

Directions:

1. Set the bones out of the chicken and cut them into one-inch pieces. Take 2 cups of chicken pieces.
2. In a large pot, add chicken broth and let it boil for 10 minutes.
3. Add noodles and vegetables to the broth.
4. Let it boil and cook for 15 minutes. Make sure noodles are tender.

5. Serve with chopped parsley on top.

Nutrition Facts Per Serving:

Calories: 569.02 kcal

Total Fat: 13.38 g

Carbs: 73.68 g

Protein: 36.8 g

Sodium: 1654.6 mg

Potassium: 1000 mg

Phosphorus: 320 mg

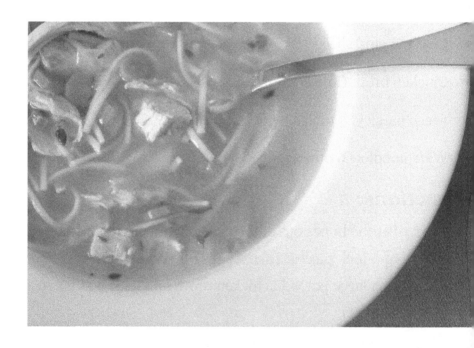

Quick and Easy Ground Beef Soup

Preparation Time: 10 minutes

Cooking Time: 1 hour

Servings: 2

Ingredients:

- Frozen mixed vegetables: 3 cups
- 1/2 cup of onion, chopped
- Beef broth (reduced-sodium): 1 cup
- White rice: 1/3 cup, uncooked
- Lemon pepper (no salt): 2 teaspoons, seasoning
- 2 cups lean ground beef
- Light or 40% fat only sour cream: 1 tablespoon
- Water: 2 cups

Directions:

1. In a pot, sauté onion, brown the beef. Drain the fat.
2. Add all the remaining ingredients and seasoning.
3. Add water and Let it boil to cook beef first for 30 minutes.
4. Lower the heat, add water, cover it and cook for 20 minutes.
5. Turn off the heat, add sour cream.

Nutrition Facts Per Serving:

Calories: 430 kcal

Protein: 20 g

Carbohydrates: 19 g

Fat: 8 g

Cholesterol: 52 mg

Sodium: 170 mg

Potassium: 448 mg

Phosphorus: 210 mg

Calcium: 43 mg

Fiber: 4.3 g

Lightning Source UK Ltd.
Milton Keynes UK
UKHW020804260821
389520UK00011B/645